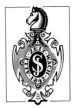

World Health Organization

The series *International Histological Classification of Tumours* consists of the following volumes. Each of these volumes – apart from volumes 1 and 2, which have already been revised – will appear in a revised edition within the next few years. Volumes of the current editions can be ordered through WHO, Distribution and Sales, Avenue Appia, CH-1211 Geneva 27.

1. Histological typing of lung tumours (1967, second edition 1981)
2. Histological typing of breast tumours (1968, second edition 1981)
3. Histological typing of soft tissue tumours (1969)
4. Histological typing of oral and oropharyngeal tumours (1971)
5. Histological typing of odontogenic tumours, jaw cysts, and allied lesions (1971)
6. Histological typing of bone tumours (1972)
7. Histological typing of salivary gland tumours (1972)
8. Cytology of the female genital tract (1973)
9. Histological typing of ovarian tumours (1973)
10. Histological typing of urinary bladder tumours (1973)
11. Histological typing of thyroid tumours (1974)
12. Histological typing of skin tumours (1974)
13. Histological typing of female genital tract tumours (1975)
14. Histological and cytological typing of neoplastic diseases of haematopoietic and lymphoid tissues (1976)
15. Histological typing of intestinal tumours (1976)
16. Histological typing of testis tumours (1977)
17. Cytology of non-gynaecological sites (1977)
18. Histological typing of gastric and oesophageal tumours (1977)
19. Histological typing of upper respiratory tract tumours (1978)
20. Histological typing of tumours of the liver, biliary tract and pancreas (1978)
21. Histological typing of tumours of the central nervous system (1979)
22. Histological typing of prostate tumours (1980)
23. Histological typing of endocrine tumours (1980)
24. Histological typing of tumours of the eye and its adnexa (1980)
25. Histological typing of kidney tumours (1981)

A coded compendium of the International Histological Classification of Tumours (1978)

In this series, colour illustrations will be limited in number in order to maintain a reasonable sales price. The present volume is an exception owing to a special subsidy obtained by the author.

A set of 92 colour slides (35 mm), corresponding to the photomicrographs in the book, is available from the American Registry of Pathology, 14th Street and Alaska Ave. NW, Washington, DC 20306, USA. For further information please see p. 67.

Histological Typing of Thyroid Tumours

Chr. Hedinger

In Collaboration with
E. D. Williams and L. H. Sobin
and Pathologists in 8 Countries

Second Edition

With 92 Figures

Springer-Verlag Berlin Heidelberg New York
London Paris Tokyo

Chr. Hedinger
Head, WHO Collaborating Centre for the
Histological Classification of Thyroid Tumours
Department of Pathology
University of Zürich, Switzerland

E. D. Williams
Head, WHO Collaborating Centre for the
Histological Classification of Endocrine Tumours
Department of Pathology
University of Wales College of Medicine
Cardiff, Wales, U. K.

L. H. Sobin
Head, WHO Collaborating Centre for the
International Histological Classification of Tumours
Armed Forces Institute of Pathology
Washington, D. C., USA

First edition published by WHO in 1974 as No. 11 in the International Histological Classification
of Tumours series

ISBN 3-540-19244-1 Springer-Verlag Berlin Heidelberg New York
ISBN 0-387-19244-1 Springer-Verlag New York Berlin Heidelberg

Library of Congress Cataloging-in-Publication Data
Hedinger, Chr. E. (Christoph Ernst), 1917–   Histological typing of thyroid tumours /
Chr. Hedinger, in collaboration with E. D. Williams and L. H. Sobin. – 2nd rev. ed.   p. cm. –
(International histological classification of tumours ; 11)
Includes index.
ISBN 0-387-19244-1 (U. S.)
1. Thyroid gland – Tumors – Histopathology – Classification. I. Williams, E. D. (Edward Dillwyn)
II. Sobin, L. H. III. Title. IV. Series: International histological classification of tumours ; no. 11.
[DNLM: 1. Thyroid Neoplasms – classification. WI IN764G v. 11a / WK 15 H454h]
RC258.I45 no. 11 1988 [RC280.T6] 616.99'207583 s – dc19 [616.99'244]
DNLM/DLC for Library of Congress   88-20186 CIP

Typesetting, printing and binding: Appl, Wemding
2121/3145-543210 – Printed on acid-free paper

General Preface to the Series

Among the prerequisites for comparative studies of cancer are international agreement on histological criteria for the definition and classification of cancer types and a standardized nomenclature. An internationally agreed classification of tumours, acceptable alike to physicians, surgeons, radiologists, pathologists and statisticians, would enable cancer workers in all parts of the world to compare their findings and would facilitate collaboration among them.

In a report published in 1952,[1] a subcommittee of the World Health Organization (WHO) Expert Committee on Health Statistics discussed the general principles that should govern the statistical classification of tumours and agreed that, to ensure the necessary flexibility and ease of coding, three separate classifications were needed according to (1) anatomical site, (2) histological type, and (3) degree of malignancy. A classification according to anatomical site is available in the International Classification of Diseases.[2]

In 1956, the WHO Executive Board passed a resolution[3] requesting the Director-General to explore the possibility that WHO might organize centres in various parts of the world and arrange for the collection of human tissues and their histological classification. The main purpose of such centres would be to develop histological definitions of cancer types and to facilitate the wide adoption of a uniform nomenclature. The resolution was endorsed by the Tenth World Health Assembly in May 1957.[4]

---

[1] WHO (1952) WHO Technical Report Series. No. 53, 1952, p 45
[2] WHO (1977) Manual of the international statistical classification of diseases, injuries, and causes of death. 1975 version Geneva
[3] WHO (1956) WHO Official Records. No. 68, p 14 (resolution EB 17. R40)
[4] WHO (1957) WHO Official Records. No. 79, p 467 (resolution WHA 10.18)

Since 1958, WHO has established a number of centres concerned with this subject. The result of this endeavour has been the International Histological Classification of Tumours, a multivolumed series whose first edition was published between 1967 and 1981. The present revised second edition aims to update the classification, reflecting progress in diagnosis and the relevance of tumour types to clinical and epidemiological features.

Preface to Histological Typing of Thyroid Tumours, Second Edition

The first edition of Histological Typing of Thyroid Tumours[1] was the result of a collaborative effort organized by WHO and carried out by the International Reference/Collaborating Centre for the Histological Classification of Thyroid Tumours at the Department of Pathology, Faculty of Medicine, University of Zürich, Switzerland. The Centre was established in 1964 and the classification was published in 1974.

In order to keep the classification up to date, a meeting was convened at the Centre in 1986 to discuss proposals for revision (participants listed on pages XI and XII). At this meeting the present classification, definitions and explanatory notes were formulated and recommended for publication.

The histological classification of thyroid tumours, which appears on page 3, contains the morphology code numbers of the International Classification of Diseases for Oncology (ICD-O)[2] and the Systematized Nomenclature of Medicine (SNOMED).[3]

It will, of course, be appreciated that the classification reflects the present state of knowledge, and modifications are almost certain to be needed as experience accumulates. Although the present classification has been adopted by the members of the group, it necessarily represents a view from which some pathologists may wish to dissent.

---

[1] Hedinger Chr, Sobin LH (1974) Histological Typing of Thyroid Tumours. Geneva, World Health Organization (International Histological Classification of Tumours, No. 11)
[2] World Health Organization (1976) International Classification of Diseases for Oncology. Geneva
[3] College of American Pathologists (1976) Systematized Nomenclature of Medicine. Chicago

It is nevertheless hoped that, in the interests of international cooperation, all pathologists will use the classification as put forward. Criticism and suggestions for its improvement will be welcomed; these should be sent to the World Health Organization, Geneva, Switzerland.

The publications in the series International Histological Classification of Tumours are not intended to serve as textbooks but rather to promote the adoption of a uniform terminology that will facilitate communication among cancer workers. For this reason the literature references have intentionally been omitted and readers should refer to standard works for bibliographies.

Table of Contents

Participants

Caillou, B., Dr.
Institut Gustave Roussy, Villejuif, France

Egloff, B., Dr.
Pathologisches Institut, Kantonsspital Winterthur, Winterthur, Switzerland (secretary of the WHO Collaborating Centre for the Histological Classification of Thyroid Tumours)

Franssila, K., Dr.
Division of Pathology, Department of Radiotherapy and Oncology, Central Hospital, Helsinki University, Helsinki, Finland

Hedinger, Chr., Dr.
Institut für Pathologie der Universität Zürich, Zürich, Switzerland (head of the WHO Collaborating Centre for the Histological Classification of Thyroid Tumours)

Khmelnitsky, O.K., Dr.
Department of Pathology, Institute for Postgraduate Medical Training, Leningrad, USSR

Lang, W., Dr.
Hannover, Federal Republic of Germany

Rosai, J., Dr.
Department of Pathology, Yale University School of Medicine, New Haven, CT, USA

Sakamoto, A., Dr.
Department of Pathology, Cancer Institute, Tokyo, Japan

Sobin, L. H., Dr.
Department of Gastrointestinal Pathology, Armed Forces Institute of Pathology, Washington, DC, USA (head of the WHO Collaborating Centre for the International Histological Classification of Tumours)

Sobrinho-Simões, M., Dr.
Department of Pathology, University of Porto, Porto, Portugal

Vickery, A. L. Jr., Dr.
Department of Pathology, Massachusetts General Hospital, Boston, MA, USA

Williams, E. D., Dr.
Department of Pathology, University of Wales College of Medicine, Cardiff, Wales, UK (head of the WHO Collaborating Centre for the Histological Classification of Endocrine Tumours)

Introduction

Knowledge of tumours of the thyroid gland has advanced considerably in the 22 years that have elapsed since work was started on the first edition of *Histological Typing of Thyroid Tumours*. In the introduction to that volume it was recognized that the definitions and classifications put forward would need revision in time, and the present text differs substantially from the first edition. As far as is possible, however, the framework of the classification proposed remains the same, as the original classification was widely accepted and proved useful in many studies.

The link between the morphological type of thyroid tumour and its epidemiology, natural history, function, prognosis and response to therapy has been further strengthened since the first edition. In particular, the decision taken to separate papillary and follicular carcinomas and exclude a mixed papillary follicular type has been well justified.

One of the major changes has been the recognition that many tumours regarded 20 years ago as small cell carcinoma were really malignant lymphoma, and this development has been incorporated into this edition, with increased importance given to primary malignant lymphoma of the thyroid. Much work has also been done on medullary carcinoma of the thyroid, its link with multiple endocrine neoplasia syndromes, and its association in its inherited form with C-cell hyperplasia; this too is recognized by an expanded section on this tumour.

Other, less frequent types of thyroid tumour have been more clearly delineated during the last 20 years; when there is sufficient evidence that the morphological type of tumour described is linked to a difference in clinical behaviour it is referred to in this volume.

A major change in the management of thyroid tumours over the last 20 years has been the introduction in many centres of fine-needle aspiration as a pre-operative diagnostic procedure, but as this technique is used for investigation rather than classification it is not illustrated in this volume.

Many problems remain unresolved and we invite the constructive criticism of all practising pathologists.

Histological Classification of Thyroid Tumours

1   Epithelial tumours

1.1   *Benign*
1.1.1 Follicular adenoma   8330/0[a]
1.1.2 Others

1.2   *Malignant*
1.2.1 Follicular carcinoma   8330/3
1.2.2 Papillary carcinoma   8260/3[b]
1.2.3 Medullary carcinoma (C-cell carcinoma)   8510/3
1.2.4 Undifferentiated (anaplastic) carcinoma   8020/3
1.2.5 Others

2   Non-epithelial tumours

3   Malignant lymphomas

4   Miscellaneous tumours

5   Secondary tumours

6   Unclassified tumours

7   Tumour-like lesions

---

[a] Morphology code of the International Classification of Diseases for Oncology (ICD-O) and the Systematized Nomenclature of Medicine (SNOMED)
[b] 8260/3 is papillary *adeno*carcinoma

Definitions and Explanatory Notes

1 Epithelial Tumours

1.1 Benign

1.1.1 Follicular Adenoma (Figs. 1–11)

A benign encapsulated tumour showing evidence of follicular cell differentiation.

The follicular adenoma is usually a solitary tumour and has a well-defined fibrous capsule. The adjacent glandular tissue may be compressed. The architectural pattern and cytological features are different from those of the surrounding gland. While these characteristics can be used to separate the typical adenoma from the typical nodule, some nodules may show one or more of these features, and distinction between the two entities may be impossible, particularly as an adenoma may arise in a nodular goitre.

Degenerative changes such as haemorrhage, oedema, fibrosis, calcification, bone formation and cyst formation may occur.

A variety of architectural patterns occurs in follicular adenomas. Any one tumour may show a uniform architecture or an admixture of two or more patterns. While the histological differences are striking, these patterns are not of any apparent clinical importance. The main patterns seen are:

Normofollicular (simple)
Macrofollicular (colloid)
Microfollicular (fetal)
Trabecular and solid (embryonal)

Among the cytological variants seen, the most important is the *follicular adenoma of oxyphilic cell type* (Fig. 4), which may show any of the above architectural patterns. These tumours are largely or entirely composed of eosinophilic cells, often with some nuclear pleomorphism and distinct nucleoli. Formerly, they were called 'Hürthle cell' adenomas (a misnomer, since what Hürthle described (in dogs) were probably parafollicular cells). Oxyphilic cells characteristically contain large numbers of mitochondria. Very rarely, cells with apparently similar light-microscope characteristics contain increased amounts of filaments, dense bodies or endoplasmic reticulum.

Several other rare cytological variants are found in follicular adenomas.

The clear cell type of follicular adenoma (Figs. 5, 6) has to be distinguished from the clear cell variant of follicular carcinoma, parathyroid adenoma or metastasis of renal carcinoma. Immunohistological methods for staining thyroglobulin are useful for the last two purposes. The clear cells contain distended and empty-looking mitochondria and/or large amounts of glycogen.

Other very rare variants of follicular adenoma consist of mucin-producing cells, lipid-rich cells or so-called signet-ring cells (Figs. 7, 8).

Some follicular adenomas with normofollicular architecture may exhibit pseudopapillary structures which can be confused with the papillae of papillary carcinoma. A number of these hyperplastic lesions are hyperfunctioning (toxic) adenomas (Fig. 11).

In some adenomas cellular proliferation is more pronounced and the architectural and cytological patterns are less regular. These tumours are referred to as *atypical adenomas* (Figs. 9, 10). In such tumours, extension through the capsule and invasion of vessels within or just outside the capsule must be carefully excluded in order to rule out the minimally invasive variant of follicular carcinoma.

1.1.2 Other Adenomas

Very rarely, salivary gland-type tumours may occur. Adenolipomas (Fig. 12) consisting of both adipose tissue and thyroid follicular cells are extremely rare, although small amounts of stromal adipocyte infiltration in follicular tumours are occasionally seen. Hyalinizing trabecular adenomas (Figs. 13, 14) are rare, but have diagnostic importance, as they may be misinterpreted as medullary or papillary carcinomas.

1.2 Malignant

1.2.1 Follicular Carcinoma (Figs. 15–32)

A malignant epithelial tumour showing evidence of follicular cell differentiation but lacking the diagnostic features of papillary carcinoma.

The morphology of follicular carcinomas is extremely variable, ranging from well-formed follicles containing colloid to a solid, cellular growth pattern. Poorly formed follicles or atypical patterns, e.g. cribriform, may occur, and coexistence of multiple architectural types is common. However, neither architectural nor cytological atypicalities are by themselves reliable criteria of malignancy, as these changes may be present in benign neoplasms, notably atypical adenomas. Mitotic activity has not proven to be a useful indicator of malignancy. Whether the usual histological growth patterns, e.g. microfollicular or trabecular, have an influence on prognosis is controversial. A group of uncommon poorly differentiated tumours with distinctive architectural features referred to as insular carcinoma is associated with a worse prognosis.

Prognostically, it is important that follicular carcinomas are classified according to their degree of invasiveness:

Minimally invasive (encapsulated) (Figs. 16, 19): Grossly encapsulated solitary tumours, often with solid, fleshy and firm cut surfaces. Minimally invasive carcinomas are almost always architecturally and cytologically indistinguishable from adenomas (viz. embryonal, fetal or atypical) and the diagnosis of malignancy depends entirely on the demonstration of unequivocal vascular invasion (often with endothelium-covered intravascular tumour masses) and/or invasion that penetrates the full thickness of the capsule. Invasion of one or more vessels within or immediately outside the capsule is present in the vast majority of cases and is a much more reliable criterion than capsular invasion. Examination of multiple blocks through the periphery of all unusually cellular encapsulated thyroid neoplasms is necessary to exclude evidence of invasion. The essentially normal survival of patients with a diagnosis of minimally invasive follicular carcinoma based on borderline histological invasion indicates the need for unequivocal evidence of invasion to establish the diagnosis of carcinoma.

Since the distinction between a minimally invasive follicular carcinoma and a follicular adenoma depends on vascular or capsular invasion, cytological studies, including aspiration cytology, may not be adequate for diagnosis. The diagnosis 'noninvasive low-grade follicular carcinoma' is not acceptable.

Widely invasive (Figs. 20, 24): These tumours show widespread infiltration of blood vessels and/or adjacent thyroid tissue and often lack complete encapsulation. In contrast to the minimally invasive tumours, they are rarely a diagnostic problem. Tumours which show extensive microscopic invasion, particularly vascular, should be placed in this category even if grossly encapsulated.

Lymph node metastases are uncommon in follicular carcinomas except in the poorly differentiated insular type. Distant metastases occur infrequently with minimally invasive carcinomas but are commonly associated with widely invasive tumours. The lungs and bones are the most frequent metastatic sites. The histology of metastases often differs from that of the primary thyroid neoplasm. Very well-differentiated metastatic carcinomas, indistinguishable from normal thyroid, were formerly called metastasizing adenoma, malignant adenoma or metastasizing goitre. The primary thyroid tumour of such cases is nearly always more cellular and less well-differentiated than the metastasis. Immunoperoxidase staining for thyroglobulin is valuable in confirming the thyroid origin of a metastatic tumour.

Variants

The *follicular carcinoma, oxyphilic cell type* (Figs. 25, 26), is largely or entirely composed of eosinophilic cells. It should not be referred to as a Hürthle cell carcinoma, a misnomer, or as an oxyphilic carcinoma, an incomplete term. The same criteria of malignancy apply to follicular tumours of oxyphilic cells as to those composed of ordinary follicular cells. Oxyphilia per se is not a criterion of malignancy. However, many tumours of oxyphilic cell type are hypercellular and all hypercellular tumours, oxyphilic or not, should be examined with more than usual care.

A rare *clear cell variant of follicular carcinoma* (Figs. 27, 28) shows similarities of architecture and clinical course to usual follicular carcinomas. These tumours must be distinguished from clear cell adenoma, parathyroid adenoma and metastatic clear cell carcinomas, particularly renal cell carcinoma. Thyroglobulin localization by immunohistochemistry is of value in the differential diagnosis.

1.2.2 Papillary Carcinoma (Figs. 33–44)

A malignant epithelial tumour showing evidence of follicular cell differentiation, typically with papillary and follicular structures as well as characteristic nuclear changes.

Less constant features of papillary carcinomas include an invasive growth pattern, psammoma bodies and a fibrous stroma. Many of these tumours lack one or more of the above features.

Most papillary carcinomas contain complex branching papillae that have a fibrovascular core covered by a single layer of tumour cells. The nuclei of papillary carcinoma cells may show a number of changes; these include: a 'ground glass' appearance, large size, pale staining, irregular outlines with deep grooves, inconspicuous nucleoli and pseudoinclusions resulting from cytoplasmic invaginations. The nuclei often overlap. These nuclear features are important in the recognition of papillary carcinoma by fine-needle aspiration cytology. Although they are helpful in establishing the diagnosis of papillary carcinoma, they are not constant and in many tumours only a minority of cells may show them.

In most papillary carcinomas, mitoses are very rare. The cytoplasm is usually pale-staining and the cells show immunohistochemical evidence of thyroglobulin production. Squamous metaplasia is sometimes present. Psammoma bodies occur in almost one half of papillary carcinomas but practically never in other thyroid lesions. Follicles are almost always present and may be the predominant component; these follicular elements are often irregularly shaped but may be well differentiated. In addition to papillary and follicular structures, solid or trabecular growth patterns may occur. Multiple microscopic tumour foci distant from the primary tumour including the contralateral lobe are often seen and in most cases are thought to represent intraglandular spread. Tumours of a mixed papillary-follicular structure exhibit the biological behaviour of papillary carcinoma and are thus classified as papillary carcinoma. 'Mixed papillary-follicular carcinoma' should not be used as a diagnostic term.

Papillary carcinomas characteristically spread to regional lymph nodes but may also metastasize to distant organs, particularly lung. The term 'lateral aberrant thyroid' should not be used. Thyroid follicles with or without papillary features in a cervical lymph node practically always represent a metastasis from a papillary thyroid carcinoma which may be clinically occult. The prognosis for intrathyroid papillary carcinoma is generally very good with or without regional lymph node metastases. The most important pathologic adverse prognostic feature is the presence of gross direct invasion of perithyroid tissues. It has been claimed that those uncommon papillary carcinomas with a trabecular growth pattern or an increased mitotic rate are associated with a less favourable prognosis. However, the value of histologic grading of papillary carcinoma remains to be substantiated.

Macropapillary structures in nodular goitre or in follicular adenoma as well as papillary infoldings in hyperplasia should not be confused with the papillae of papillary carcinoma. While the nuclear features of papillary carcinoma may be helpful in making this distinction, the other histologic features of papillary carcinoma should also be taken into consideration. Nuclear features alone, particularly pale-staining, should not be considered specific for the diagnosis of papillary carcinoma, as many of these features may be seen in a number of benign thyroid lesions. Laminated, basophilic, sometimes calcified, intrafollicular structures, apparently arising from a degenerative change in thyroid colloid, may be present in follicular adenomas or carcinomas, particularly in oxyphilic tumours. These should not be confused with true psammoma bodies, which are laminated, basophilic, calcified, stromal structures, arising from degenerative changes in the papillae of papillary carcinoma.

Variants

Papillary Microcarcinoma (Fig. 38). Papillary microcarcinoma is here defined as a papillary carcinoma 1.0 cm or less in diameter. These microcarcinomas are common in population-based autopsy studies and as incidental findings in carefully examined resected thyroid glands. Although they may be associated with cervical lymph node metastasis, the prognosis is excellent and distant metastases are exceptionally rare.

Encapsulated Variant (Fig. 40). Although most papillary carcinomas show an invasive growth pattern (Fig. 39), circumscribed or encapsulated tumours also occur, but are rare. Encapsulated papillary carcinomas may metastasize but have been reported to have an even better prognosis than the more common nonencapsulated tumours. There are no reliable morphological criteria to differentiate those associated with metastasis from those that are not. Therefore the use of the term 'papillary adenoma' is not recommended.

Follicular Variant (Fig. 41). Papillary carcinomas may be composed entirely or almost entirely of follicles. When such tumours are circumscribed their differentiation from follicular carcinomas or adenomas may be difficult. Apart from the absence of papillae these tumours resemble papillary carcinoma in their morphological features as well as their clinical behaviour.

Diffuse Sclerosing Variant (Figs. 43, 44). Rare papillary carcinomas show diffuse involvement of one or both thyroid lobes, with dense sclerosis and abundant psammoma bodies intermixed with islands of papillary carcinoma. Foci of squamous metaplasia are often seen and patchy lymphocytic infiltrates may be present. The tumour occurs mostly in young individuals. It has been suggested that this tumour has a less favourable prognosis than papillary carcinoma in general.

Oxyphilic cell type (Fig. 42). A small minority of tumours with classical papillary architecture are composed entirely of oxyphilic cells. Their nuclei generally resemble the nuclei seen in other oxyphilic tumours and do not show the nuclear changes commonly associated with papillary carcinoma. In other respects they resemble typical papillary carcinomas in both morphology and behaviour. Care should be taken to distinguish encapsulated oxyphilic follicular tumours, which often show macropapillary structures and intracolloid psammoma-like bodies, from the rare true papillary carcinoma, oxyphilic cell type.

1.2.3 Medullary Carcinoma (C-Cell Carcinoma) (Figs. 45–56)

A malignant tumour showing evidence of C-cell differentiation.

Typically it is composed of solid sheets, islands or trabeculae of polygonal or spindle-shaped cells with abundant granular cytoplasm which contains immunoreactive calcitonin.

This tumour may show a wide variety of architectural patterns and may mimic the pattern of any other type of thyroid carcinoma. Glandular, papillary, small cell and anaplastic variants have been described. Stromal amyloid is present in most tumours and is helpful but not essential for the diagnosis. The amyloid may be associated with a giant cell response, and is similar on haematoxylin-eosin (H&E) and Congo Red staining to other types of amyloid. Cytologically, the tumour cells are polygonal with an abundant granular cytoplasm, although spindle cell forms, often packeted, may occur. Nuclei are commonly regular; occasional large nuclei are not necessarily a sign of a poor prognosis. Pseudoglandular and pseudopapillary structures may be seen; occasionally true glands and more rarely true papillae may be found in part or all of the tumour. The polygonal cells of tumours with little mitotic activity commonly contain abundant immunoreactive calcitonin, although the amount may be variable from cell to cell; they are generally argyrophilic. Tumours with a high mitotic rate, often predominantly of the spindle cell type, tend to have a poor prognosis; they may show less strong immunoreactivity for calcitonin, but are usually strongly positive for carcinoembryonic antigen.

Medullary carcinoma may produce a wide variety of peptides; occasionally mucin is produced, and some tumours contain melanin. Calcitonin is always produced, while other peptides, such as adrenocorticotrophic hormone (ACTH), are secreted by only some tumours. Diarrhoea and Cushing's syndrome are the two most important humorally mediated clinical conditions associated with this tumour.

While the range of architectural patterns and of degrees of differentiation seen in medullary carcinoma is important diagnostically, different areas within one tumour may show different features. Formal classification into multiple different sub-types is not recommended.

Inherited Medullary Carcinoma and C-cell Hyperplasia

A minority of medullary carcinomas are genetically determined, when they may be associated with phaeochromocytomas or other lesions. In genetically determined cases the tumour is commonly bilateral and arises in a background of pre-existing hyperplasia of C-cells; this feature may be seen in the thyroid bordering the tumour (Figs. 55, 56). Children or young adults carrying the gene for inherited medullary carcinoma may on thyroidectomy show only C-cell hyperplasia, diffuse or nodular, without overt malignancy.

The hyperplasia is not uniform throughout the thyroid gland but is usually found in the central part of each lateral lobe, over a rather larger area than is the case for normal C cells. It may be diffuse or nodular; the nodules are usually multiple and rounded, lack amyloid, often contain some surviving thyroid follicles, and show slightly more pleomorphism than normal C cells. C-cell identification on H&E stained sections is not reliable and a special technique such as calcitonin immunolocalization should be used.

Variant
Mixed Medullary-Follicular Carcinoma. This tumour shows both the morphological features of medullary carcinoma together with immunoreactive calcitonin, and the morphological features of follicular carcinoma together with immunoreactive thyroglobulin. Such tumours are rare and of uncertain histogenesis. The presence of entrapped thyroid follicles in primary medullary carcinomas, usually at the periphery of the tumour, should not be mistaken for neoplastic follicular cell differentiation. The presence of immunoreactive thyroglobulin in the cells of medullary carcinoma in the immediate vicinity of trapped thyroid follicles may be due to an artifact or to uptake of thyroglobulin by these cells rather than their synthesis of thyroglobulin. Absolute proof of the occurrence of this lesion depends on identification of both patterns of differentiation in metastatic tumours. The presence of immunoreactive thyroglobulin in medullary carcinoma cells without structural evidence of follicular differentiation is not regarded as sufficient for the diagnosis of mixed medullary-follicular carcinoma.

1.2.4 Undifferentiated (Anaplastic) Carcinoma (Figs. 57–69)

A highly malignant tumour composed in part or wholly of undifferentiated cells.

Definite epithelial neoplastic structures are usually present, although examination of multiple sections, the use of immunohistochemical stains for epithelial markers or electron microscopy may be necessary for confirmation. The tumour is typically composed of varying proportions of spindle, polygonal and giant cells; such tumours may resemble a sarcoma. Tumours previously called small cell undifferentiated carcinomas are now recognized to be, for the most part, malignant lymphomas. The term 'small cell undifferentiated carcinoma' should only be used if a malignant lymphoma, a medullary or follicular carcinoma composed largely of small cells, or a metastasis can be excluded. The application of immunohistochemical methods may be necessary.

Many of the undifferentiated tumours are considered to represent the terminal stage in the dedifferentiation of a follicular or papillary carcinoma, because of the presence of a residual well-differentiated component. Tumours combining obvious papillary or follicular carcinoma with undifferentiated carcinoma should be reported as undifferentiated carcinomas, although the proportions of the differentiated and undifferentiated elements should be indicated. In cases with very small undifferentiated foci in an otherwise well-differentiated carcinoma the prognosis seems to be somewhat better than in cases with an extensive undifferentiated component.

In undifferentiated carcinomas there is often a mixture of components. These may include squamous cells, osteoclast-like giant cells and sarcomatous foci such as fibrosarcoma, malignant fibrous histiocytoma, osteosarcoma, chondrosarcoma, leiomyosarcoma, rhabdomyosarcoma or haemangioendothelioma. If epithelial elements can be demonstrated, these tumours should be classified as undifferentiated carcinoma even in the presence of areas with specific sarcomatous differentiation rather than as carcinosarcoma.

In some primary undifferentiated malignant tumours detailed studies of multiple blocks fail to show any signs of epithelial or unequivocal sarcomatous differentiation. It is suggested that, because of their similarity to tumours in which an epithelial component can be demonstrated, the tradition of placing these tumours in the same category as undifferentiated carcinomas be continued. They could be reported as 'undifferentiated malignant tumour, probably undifferentiated carcinoma'. The prognosis of these lesions is the same as that of the typical undifferentiated carcinoma of the thyroid.

1.2.5 Other Carcinomas

This category comprises an extremely rare group of carcinomas characterized by the presence of mucin-producing cells, keratin, or both, and lacking the typical features of the above major tumour types. These tumours have been referred to as mucinous carcinoma, squamous cell carcinoma and mucoepidermoid carcinoma, respectively. It is not clear whether they represent separate entities or are the expression of metaplastic changes.

The term 'squamous cell carcinoma' (Fig. 70) should be reserved for tumours composed entirely of cells showing so-called intercellular bridges and/or forming keratin. Such a tumour should be distinguished from direct extension from primary carcinomas of the larynx, trachea, or oesophagus, metastases from a distant site, and squamous metaplastic changes occurring in papillary carcinoma or thyroiditis. Largely undifferentiated malignant tumours containing a squamous component should be classified under the category of undifferentiated carcinoma.

2 Non-epithelial Tumours (Figs. 71–74)

Benign non-epithelial tumours are very rare. They are classified according to the WHO Histological Typing of Soft-Tissue Tumours.

Sarcomas of the thyroid are also very rare (Figs. 71, 72). In general there is nothing to distinguish thyroid sarcomas from those of other organs. Since undifferentiated carcinomas may resemble spindle cell sarcomas, and may show a variety of sarcomatous differentiation, it is often difficult or impossible to distinguish thyroid sarcomas from undifferentiated carcinomas. From a practical standpoint, sarcoma-like tumours of the thyroid should be regarded as undifferentiated carcinomas in the absence of indisputable proof to the contrary. The diagnosis of sarcoma should only be made in tumours lacking all evidence of epithelial differentiation (co-existence of better differentiated epithelial components, squamous foci, unequivocal epithelial features at the ultrastructural level or positive immunoreactivity for cytokeratin) and showing definite evidence of specific sarcomatous differentiation.

The *malignant haemangioendothelioma* (Figs. 73, 74) is a rare, distinctive, highly malignant tumour developing in most instances in a long-standing nodular goitre. Extensive necrosis and haemorrhage are typical. In the peripheral areas there are loose strands and vascular-like clefts lined by tumour cells which exhibit light-microscopic, ultrastructural and immunohistochemical features of endothelial cells. It is almost exclusively found in populations in mountainous areas, especially in central Europe. If epithelial differentiation is present the tumour is classified as an undifferentiated carcinoma.

3 Malignant Lymphomas (Figs. 75, 76)

Malignant lymphomas can involve the thyroid as the only manifestation of the disease or as part of systemic spread. The majority of primary thyroid lymphomas arise on a background of chronic thyroiditis. Cases of thyroid lymphoma have often been misdiagnosed in the past as small cell carcinoma of diffuse type, mainly because of entrapment of follicles and 'packing' of their lumina by tumour cells. Staining for leucocyte common antigen or similar antigens is usually positive in malignant lymphoma, and is therefore of use in the differential diagnosis. Tumour extension outside the thyroid capsule is associated with an unfavourable prognosis. If dissemination occurs, involvement of the gastrointestinal tract is often a feature.

The large majority of thyroid lymphomas are of non-Hodgkin's type and should be classified using the same terminology as is applied to lymphoid tissues. Most are of the diffuse, large, non-cleaved (centroblastic) type, a B-cell malignancy of follicular centre cell derivation. The second most common form is the immunoblastic type, sometimes exhibiting prominent plasmacytoid features. Cases of primary plasmacytomas of the thyroid have also been reported.

4 Miscellaneous Tumours

Parathyroid tissue can occasionally be found within the thyroid gland. Normal parathyroid tissue is usually easily distinguished from thyroid tissue but intrathyroid parathyroid lesions, especially adenomas with follicular structures or oncocytic changes, may pose diagnostic problems.

Paragangliomas identical to those occuring in the carotid body can exceptionally be found within the thyroid, sometimes in association with paragangliomas at other sites (Figs. 77, 78). They can resemble medullary carcinomas with a nesting configuration of the tumour cells.

A very rare and unusual thyroid tumour of young individuals composed of an admixture of spindle-shaped (keratin-positive) epithelial cells and well-differentiated mucin-producing glandular structures has been described as 'spindle cell tumour with mucous cysts'. This is a low-grade malignancy of obscure histogenesis which should be distinguished from undifferentiated carcinoma and malignant teratoma.

Exceptionally, teratomas can be seen in or adjacent to the thyroid. Most of them occur in the newborn and are usually benign.

Tumours with features of carcinosarcoma are classified as undifferentiated carcinoma (see discussion under 'Undifferentiated Carcinoma').

5 Secondary Tumours (Figs. 79–82)

Microscopic metastases to the thyroid are common findings in carefully studied autopsies of patients with malignant tumours, particularly malignant melanomas and carcinomas of lung and breast. They are however rarely a cause of clinical thyroid enlargement. While any carcinoma may present in this way, renal cell carcinoma shows a particular predilection for large clinically solitary thyroid metastases. These may simulate a primary thyroid neoplasm both clinically and pathologically, often showing one or several sharply limited tumours that may have a central hyalinized scar and histologically resemble clear cell follicular carcinoma or adenoma. Staining for thyroglobulin can help distinguish these tumours from primary clear cell tumours of the thyroid. The majority of thyroid tumours composed solely of clear cells appear to be metastases. The thyroid may be involved by direct extension from head-and-neck tumours including pharyngeal, laryngeal and oesophageal squamous cell carcinomas.

6 Unclassified Tumours

Benign or malignant tumours that cannot be placed in any of the categories described above.

7 Tumour-like Lesions

Hyperplastic goitres (Figs. 83–88), both diffuse and nodular [e.g. Graves' disease (Basedow's disease), endemic goitre and dyshormonogenetic goitres], often exhibit areas of follicular proliferation with infoldings which may simulate neoplastic papillae. The macropapillary structures of nodular hyperplasia may also be confused with papillary carcinoma. Hyperplastic nodular goitres often contain encapsulated adenoma-like lesions with atypical cellularity and irregularity of outline at the capsular margin suggesting the diagnosis of follicular carcinoma. The adenomatous goitre of dyshormonogenesis may be particularly difficult to distinguish from malignancy. Carcinoma, however, is rarely associated with dyshormonogenetic goitres.

Thyroid cysts usually represent degenerative change and old haemorrhage within nodules or adenomas. Rarely epithelial-lined cysts may be found. Since cancers, particularly papillary, may also be cystic, all cystic lesions should be carefully examined.

Solid cell nests (Fig. 89) are a normal finding and may resemble foci of squamous metaplasia. They frequently contain acid mucin. C cells are commonly found in the vicinity of such cell nests.

Ectopic thyroid tissue (Fig. 90) is found in a midline location from the base of the tongue into the mediastinum. In addition, islands of normal or nodular thyroid tissue separated from the thyroid gland are occasionally found in the soft tissues of the neck. These should not be misinterpreted as metastases from a thyroid carcinoma. Such lesions may follow surgery or other trauma, or may represent sequestration of thyroid tissue, usually from nodular goitres.

Lymph nodes removed in neck dissections for non-thyroid diseases may show microscopic foci of apparently normal thyroid follicles. The great majority of these are metastatic from clinically occult papillary carcinomas.

In *chronic thyroiditis,* particularly of the *Hashimoto type,* some changes may be mistaken for malignancy. The heavy lymphoid infiltration may suggest malignant lymphoma. In some cases the epithelial proliferation is prominent and may imitate a carcinoma. Thyroiditis presenting in small biopsies of the thyroid or in sequestered thyroid tissue may lead to an erroneous diagnosis of metastatic thyroid carcinoma in a lymph node.

Riedel's thyroiditis, a very rare disease, is a unique inflammatory proliferative fibrotic lesion often associated with an occlusive phlebitis. It is important because of its tendency to invade both thyroid and perithyroidal tissue simulating a malignant process.

In a wide variety of thyroid diseases, *pleomorphic follicular cells* may be mistaken for evidence of malignancy. These cells are characterized by large and often bizarre hyperchromatic nuclei. They may occur in hyperplasia, chronic thyroiditis, and in glands which have been submitted to external irradiation or radioiodine.

A firm, enlarged thyroid may result from *primary or secondary amyloidosis* – amyloid goitre (Figs. 91, 92) – and may be associated with deposits of fatty tissue.

Subject Index

Unless otherwise stated, all the preparations shown in the photomicrographs reproduced on the following pages were stained with haematoxylin-eosin.

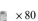

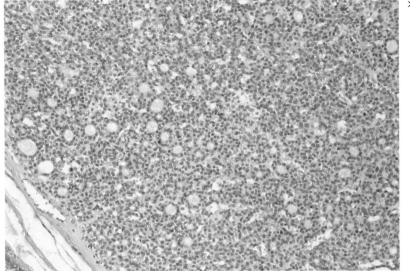

Fig. 1. *Follicular adenoma*

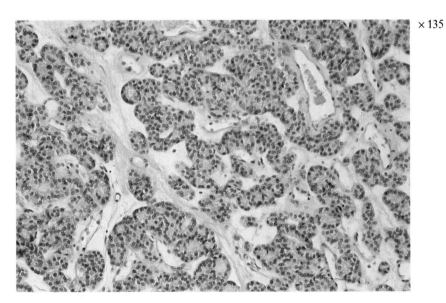

Fig. 2. *Follicular adenoma*, microfollicular

22

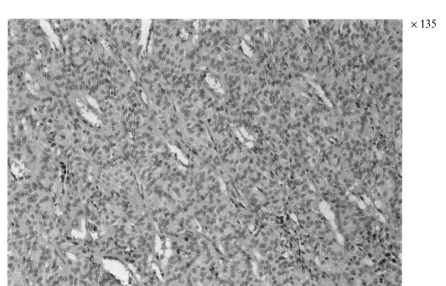

×135

Fig. 3. *Follicular adenoma*, trabecular pattern

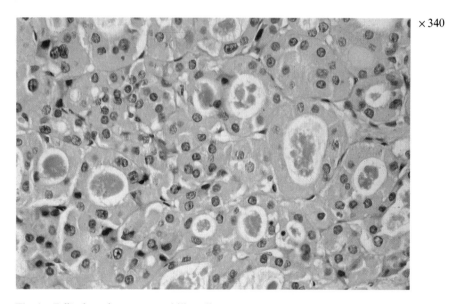

×340

Fig. 4. *Follicular adenoma*, oxyphilic cell type

× 340

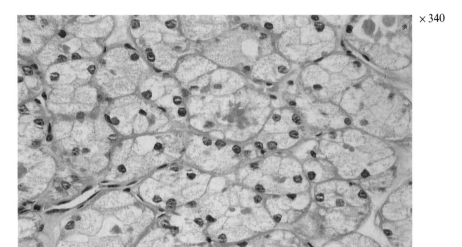

Fig. 5. *Follicular adenoma,* clear cell type

× 340

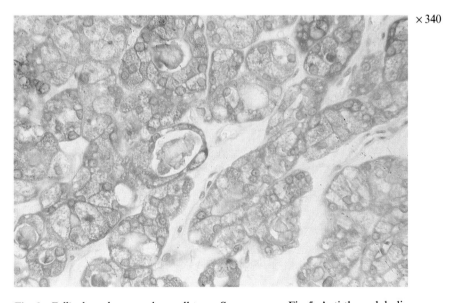

Fig. 6. *Follicular adenoma,* clear cell type. Same case as Fig. 5. Anti-thyroglobulin

24

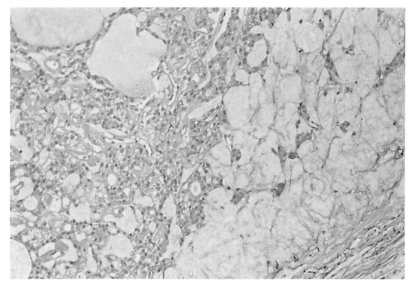

Fig. 7. *Follicular adenoma*, mucin producing. Alcian blue stain

×135

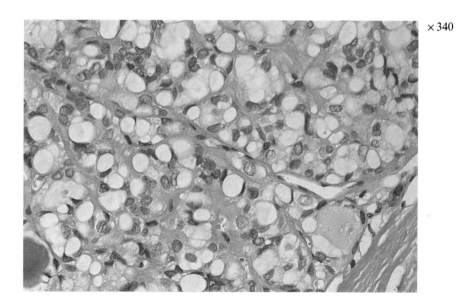

Fig. 8. *Follicular adenoma* with signet-ring cells

×340

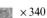

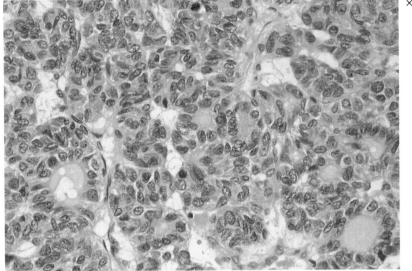

Fig. 9. *Atypical adenoma.* Considerable proliferation

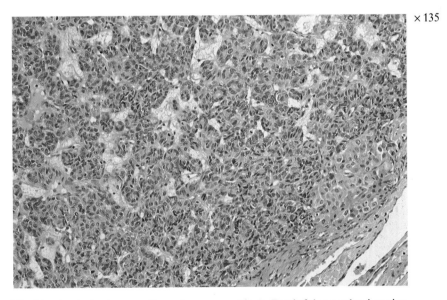

Fig. 10. *Atypical adenoma.* Same tumour as Fig. 9. Doubtful capsular invasion *(bottom right)*

× 135

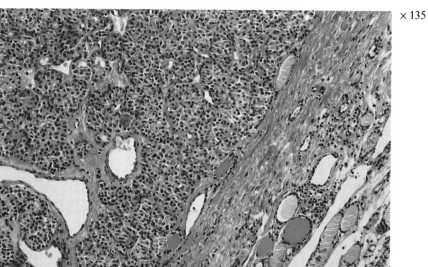

Fig. 11. *Follicular adenoma* with signs of hyperfunction (so-called toxic adenoma). Atrophy of adjacent thyroid tissue

× 135

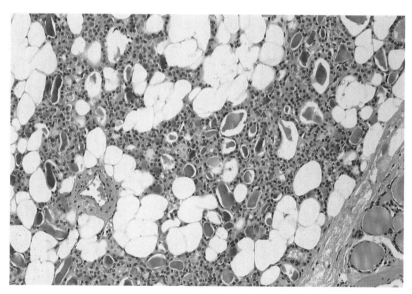

Fig. 12. *Adenolipoma*

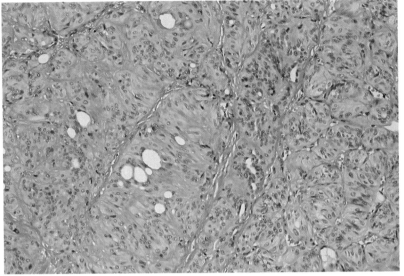

Fig. 13. *Hyalinizing trabecular adenoma*

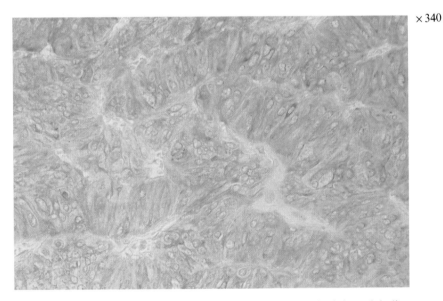

Fig. 14. *Hyalinizing trabecular adenoma*. Same case as Fig. 13. Anti-thyroglobulin

× 340

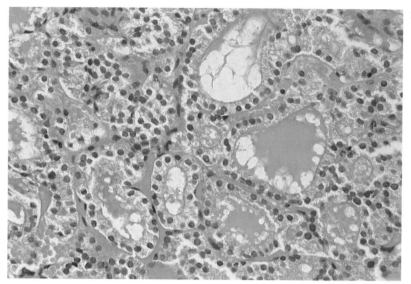

Fig. 15. *Follicular carcinoma*, bone metastasis. Well-formed follicles. Same case as Figs. 16 and 17

× 135

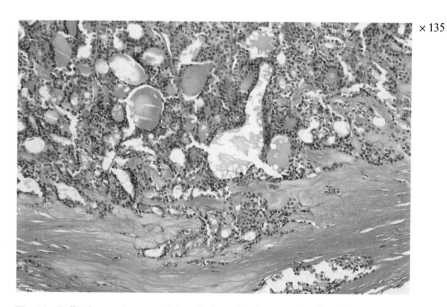

Fig. 16. *Follicular carcinoma*, minimally invasive (encapsulated). Primary tumour of Fig. 15

× 340

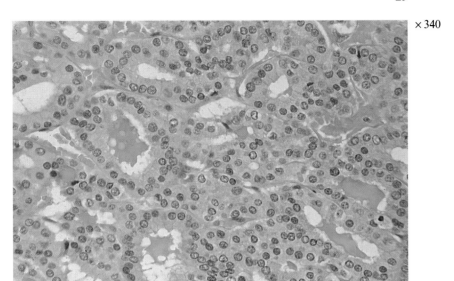

Fig. 17. *Follicular carcinoma.* Same tumour as Fig. 16

× 135

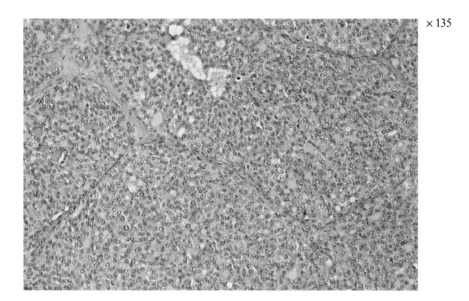

Fig. 18. *Follicular carcinoma.* Follicular and trabecular pattern

30

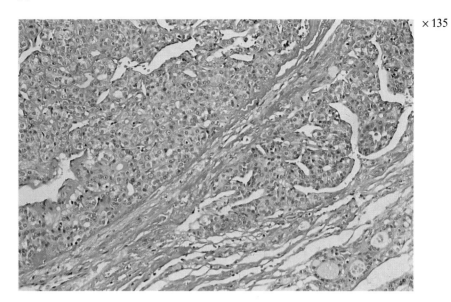

× 135

Fig. 19. *Follicular carcinoma*, minimally invasive. Capsular invasion

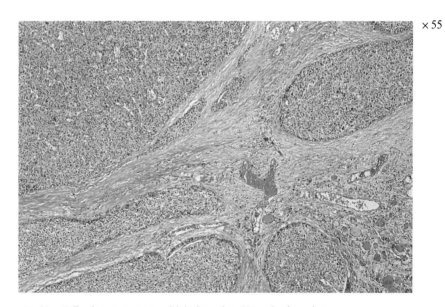

× 55

Fig. 20. *Follicular carcinoma*, widely invasive. Vascular invasion

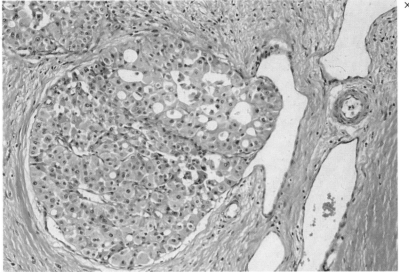

Fig. 21. *Follicular carcinoma.* Vascular invasion in capsular region

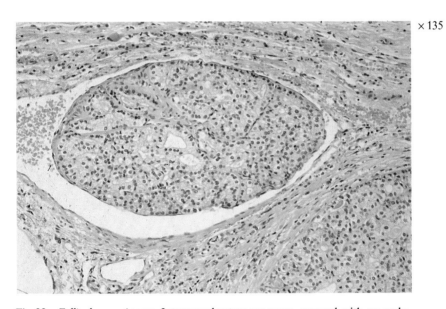

Fig. 22. *Follicular carcinoma.* Intravascular tumour mass, covered with an endo-thelial layer

32

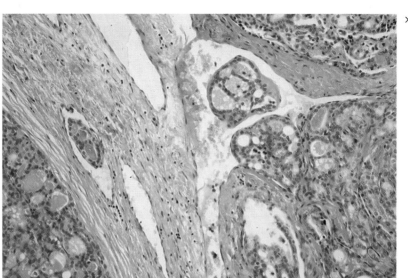

×135

Fig. 23. *Follicular carcinoma*. Vascular invasion in centre of the tumour. Intravascular endothelium-covered tumour masses

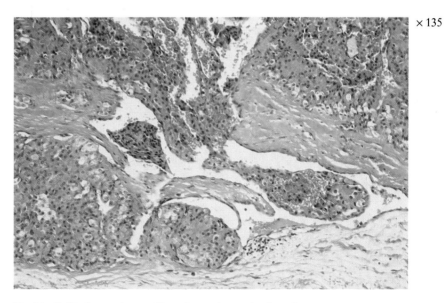

×135

Fig. 24. *Follicular carcinoma*. Capsular and vascular invasion

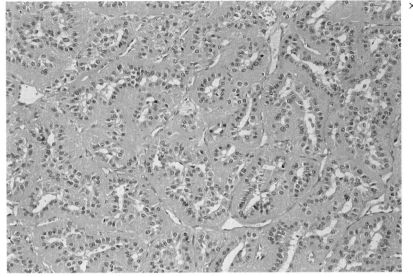

×135

Fig. 25. *Follicular carcinoma,* oxyphilic cell type

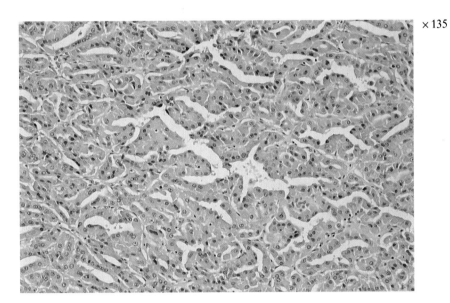

×135

Fig. 26. *Follicular carcinoma,* oxyphilic cell type. Pseudopapillary structures

34

×340

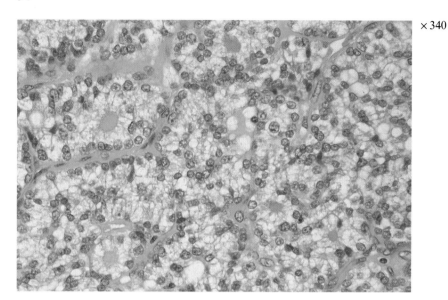

Fig. 27. *Follicular carcinoma,* clear cell variant

×340

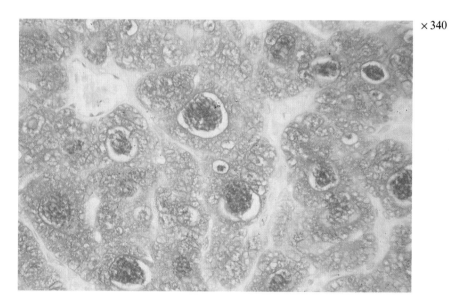

Fig. 28. *Follicular carcinoma,* clear cell variant. Same case as Fig. 27. Anti-thyro-globulin

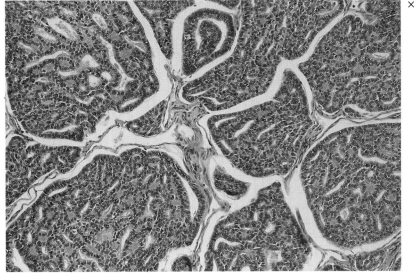

Fig. 29. *Follicular carcinoma,* so-called insular variant

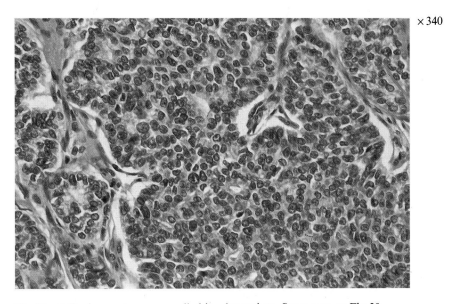

Fig. 30. *Follicular carcinoma,* so-called insular variant. Same case as Fig. 29

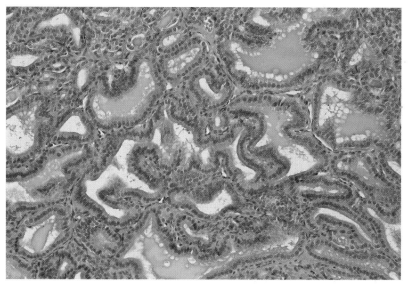

× 135

Fig. 31. *Follicular carcinoma,* pseudopapillary formation. Not to be misinterpreted as papillary carcinoma

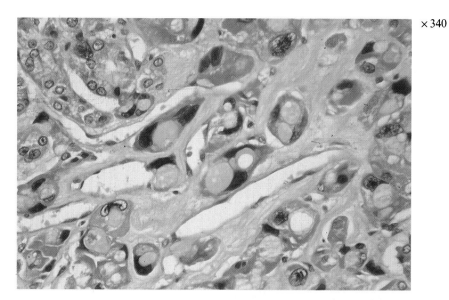

× 340

Fig. 32. *Follicular carcinoma,* degenerated follicular cells. Not to be interpreted as a sign of an undifferentiated carcinoma

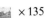

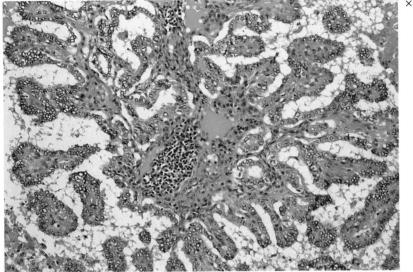

Fig. 33. *Papillary carcinoma.* Papillae with fibrous stroma

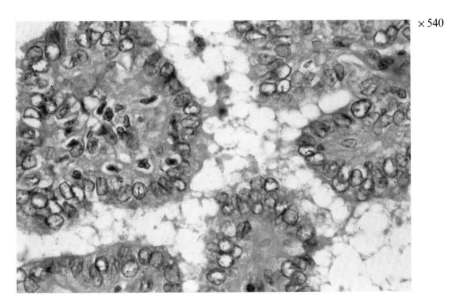

Fig. 34. *Papillary carcinoma.* Overlapping so-called ground-glass nuclei with nuclear grooves

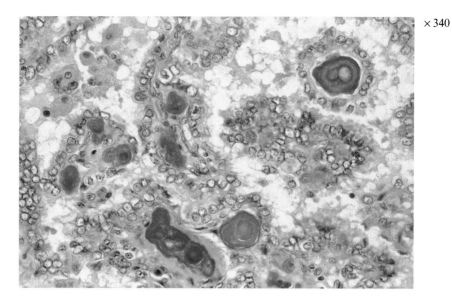

×340

Fig. 35. *Papillary carcinoma.* Psammoma bodies

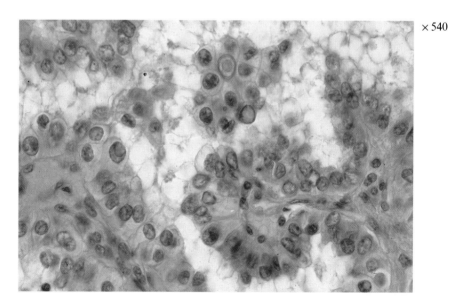

×540

Fig. 36. *Papillary carcinoma.* Nuclear pseudoinclusions resulting from cytoplasmic invagination

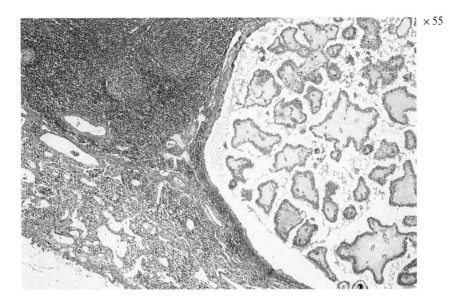

×55

Fig. 37. *Papillary carcinoma.* Cystic lymph node metastasis

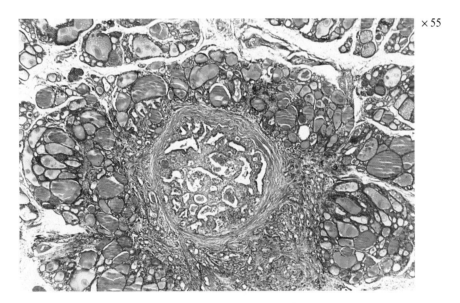

×55

Fig. 38. *Papillary microcarcinoma,* partially encapsulated

40

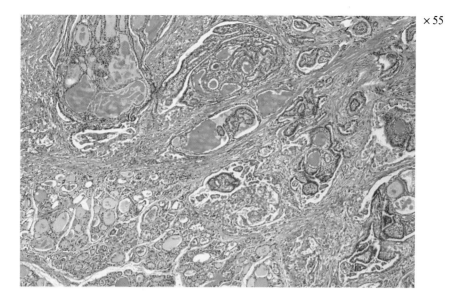

Fig. 39. *Papillary carcinoma,* widely invasive

×55

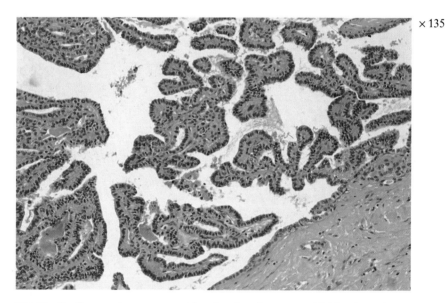

Fig. 40. *Papillary carcinoma,* encapsulated variant (compare with Figs. 85 and 86)

×135

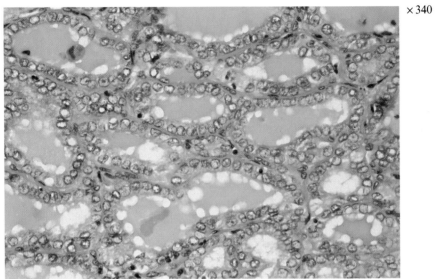

Fig. 41. *Papillary carcinoma*, follicular variant

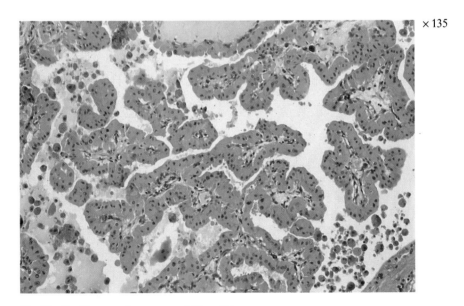

Fig. 42. *Papillary carcinoma*, oxyphilic cell type

42

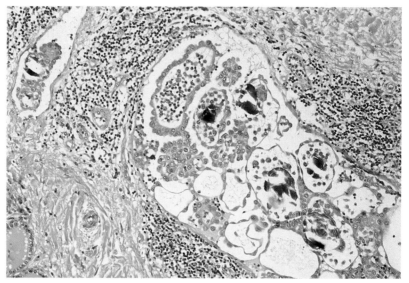

Fig. 43. *Papillary carcinoma*, diffuse sclerosing variant. 15-year-old girl

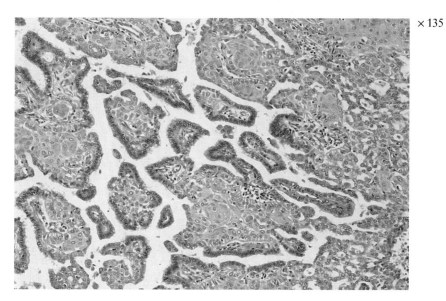

Fig. 44. *Papillary carcinoma*, diffuse sclerosing variant with squamous metaplasia. 14-year-old boy

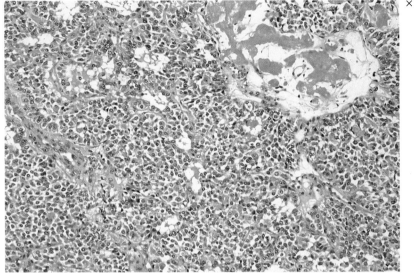

Fig. 45. *Medullary carcinoma,* small cell carcinoid-like pattern

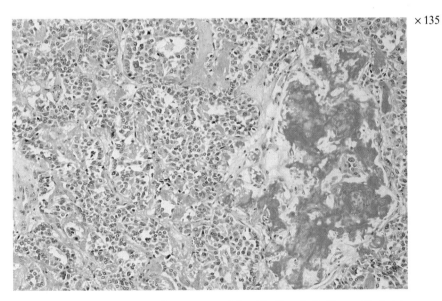

Fig. 46. *Medullary carcinoma.* Same case as Figs. 45, 47 and 48. Congo Red stain of amyloid deposits

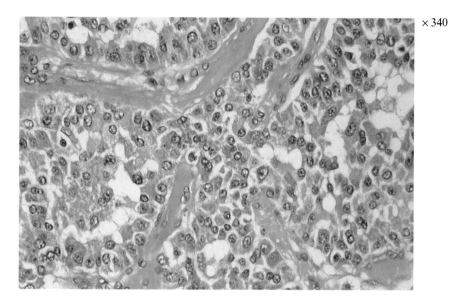

×340

Fig. 47. *Medullary carcinoma.* Same case as Figs. 45, 46 and 48, higher magnification

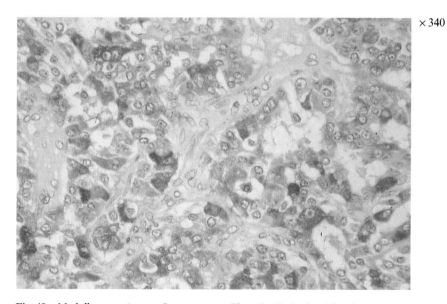

×340

Fig. 48. *Medullary carcinoma.* Same case as Figs. 45–47. Anti-calcitonin

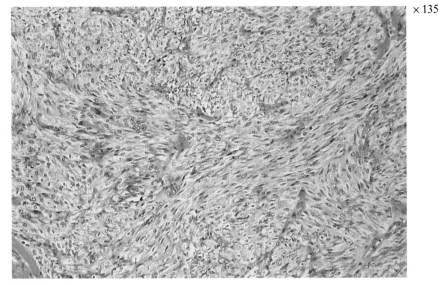

Fig. 49. *Medullary carcinoma, spindle cell pattern*

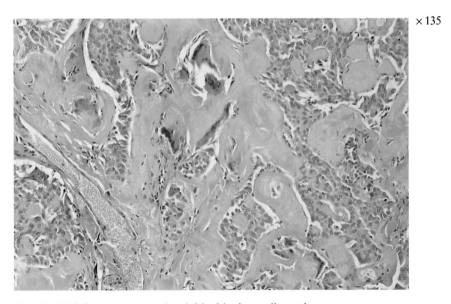

Fig. 50. *Medullary carcinoma.* Amyloid with giant cell reaction

46

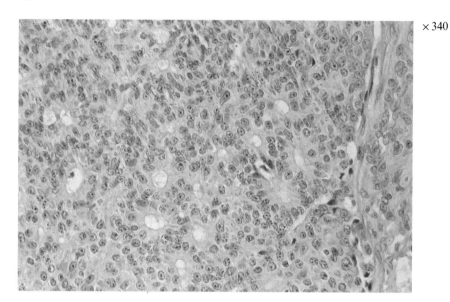

×340

Fig. 51. *Medullary carcinoma* with glandular structures

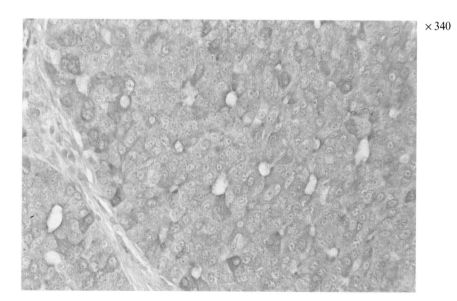

×340

Fig. 52. *Medullary carcinoma*. Same case as Fig. 51. Anti-calcitonin

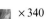

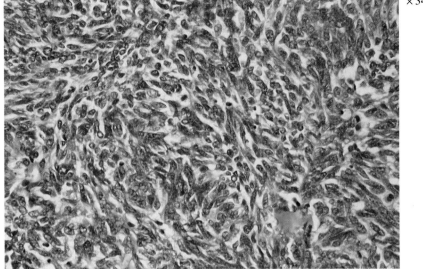

Fig. 53. *Medullary carcinoma,* poorly differentiated, spindle cell pattern

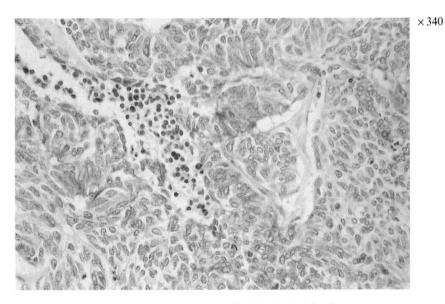

Fig. 54. *Medullary carcinoma.* Same case as Fig. 53. Anti-calcitonin

48

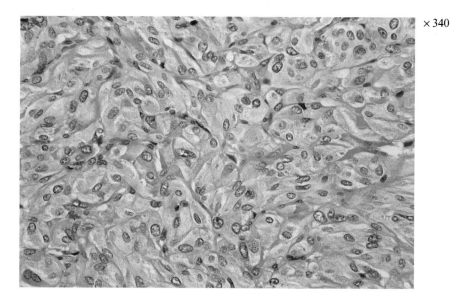

×340

Fig. 55. *Inherited medullary carcinoma.* Patient with multiple endocrine neoplasia (MEN) Type II

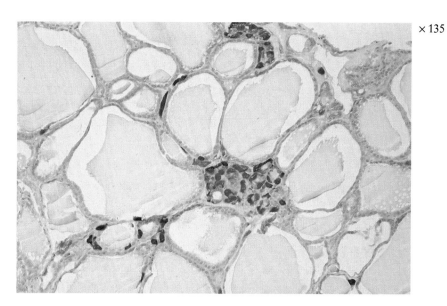

×135

Fig. 56. *Inherited medullary carcinoma.* Same case as Fig. 55. Hyperplasia of C cells in tumour-free thyroid tissue. Anti-calcitonin

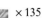

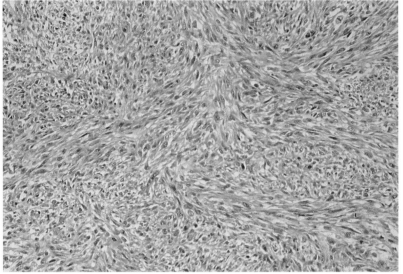

Fig. 57. *Undifferentiated carcinoma.* Spindle cells

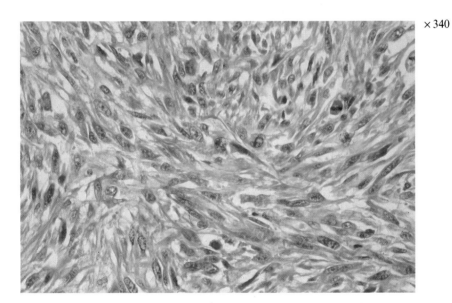

Fig. 58. *Undifferentiated carcinoma.* Spindle cells. Same tumour as Fig. 57

50

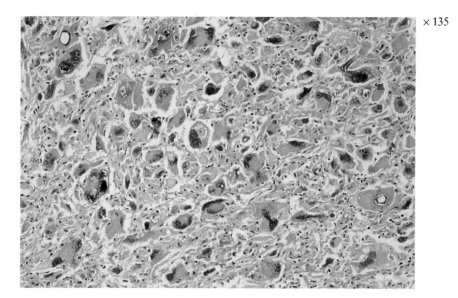

×135

Fig. 59. *Undifferentiated carcinoma*. Polygonal and giant cells

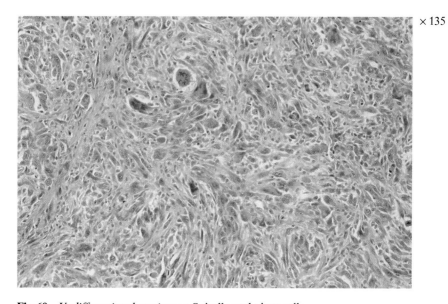

×135

Fig. 60. *Undifferentiated carcinoma*. Spindle and giant cells

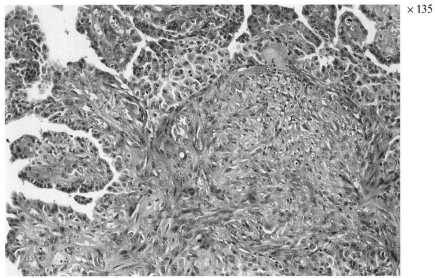

Fig. 61. *Undifferentiated carcinoma.* Residual papillary carcinoma

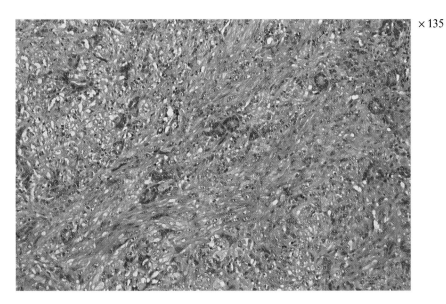

Fig. 62. *Undifferentiated carcinoma.* Residual follicular carcinoma

52

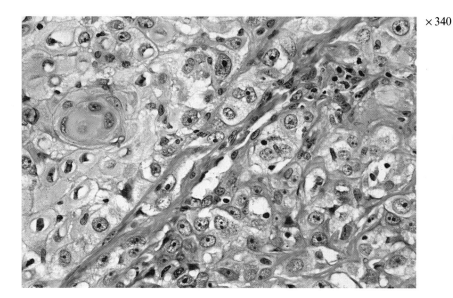 ×340

Fig. 63. *Undifferentiated carcinoma.* Squamous metaplasia

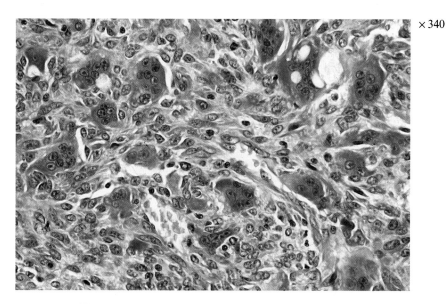 ×340

Fig. 64. *Undifferentiated carcinoma.* Osteoclast-like elements

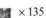

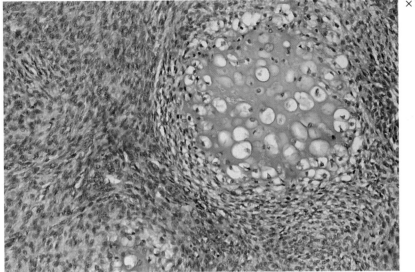

Fig. 65. *Undifferentiated carcinoma.* Chondrosarcoma-like focus

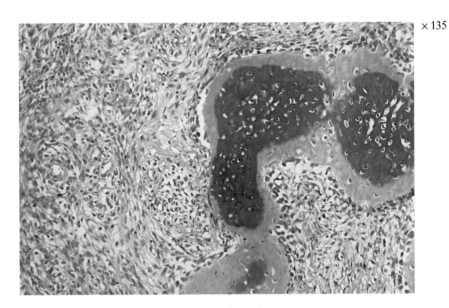

Fig. 66. *Undifferentiated carcinoma.* Bone formation

54

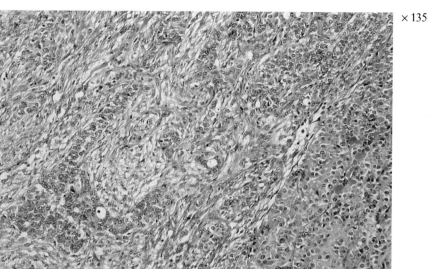

×135

Fig. 67. *Undifferentiated carcinoma.* Follicular structures and rhabdomyosarcomatous foci (see Fig. 68)

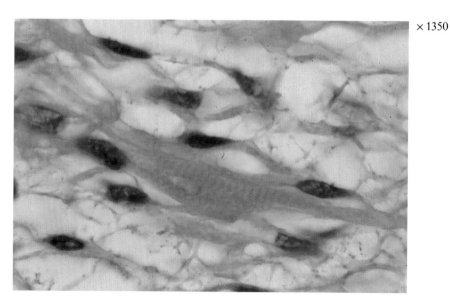

×1350

Fig. 68. *Undifferentiated carcinoma.* Same case as Fig. 67. Rhabdomyosarcomatous elements

×340

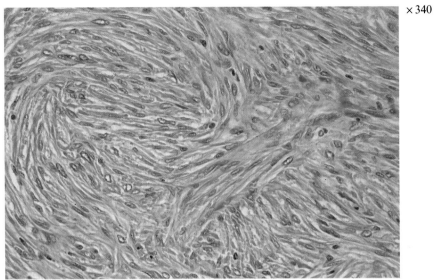

Fig. 69. *Undifferentiated carcinoma.* Malignant fibrous histiocytoma-like pattern

×340

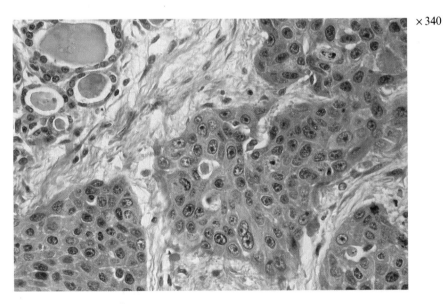

Fig. 70. *Squamous cell carcinoma*

56

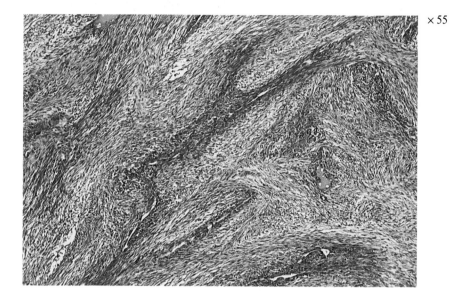

×55

Fig. 71. *Fibrosarcoma*

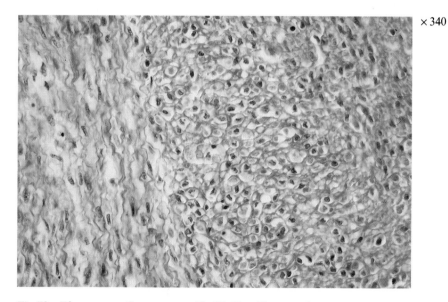

×340

Fig. 72. *Fibrosarcoma.* Same case as Fig. 71. Van Gieson stain

× 135

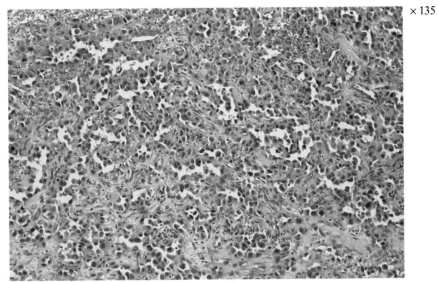

Fig. 73. *Malignant haemangioendothelioma*

× 340

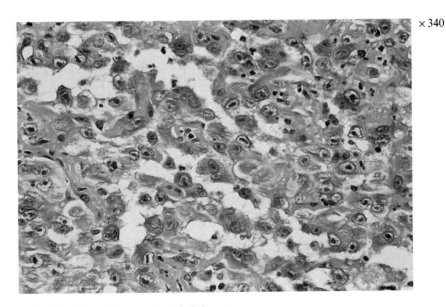

Fig. 74. *Malignant haemangioendothelioma*

58

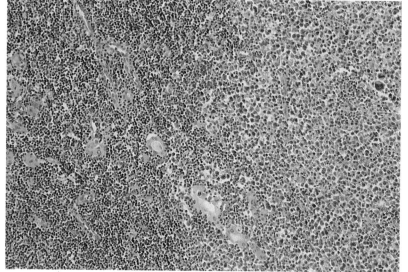

×135

Fig. 75. *Malignant lymphoma* (right) and *chronic thyroiditis* (left)

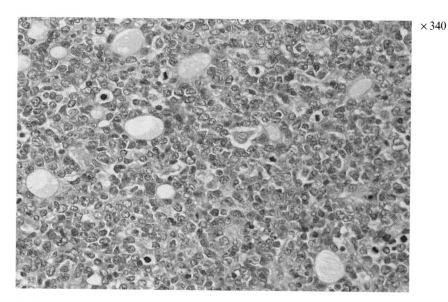

×340

Fig. 76. *Malignant lymphoma*, diffuse large non-cleaved (centroblastic) type. Residual follicles invaded by tumour cells

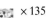

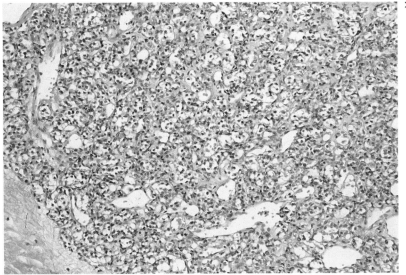

Fig. 77. *Intrathyroid paraganglioma*

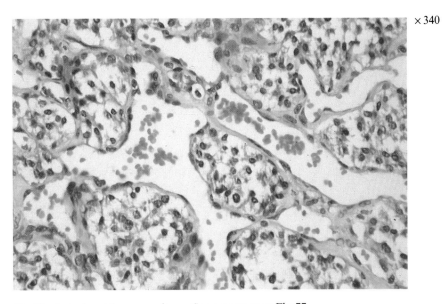

Fig. 78. *Intrathyroid paraganglioma.* Same tumour as Fig. 77

60

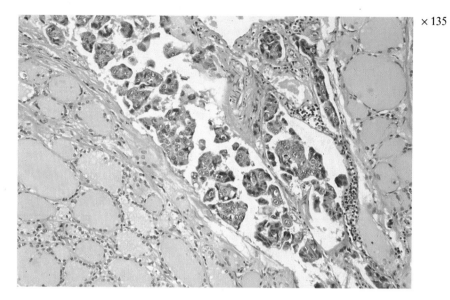

×135

Fig. 79. *Metastasis* of a papillary carcinoma of the lung

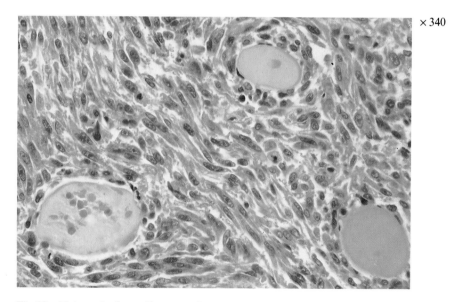

×340

Fig. 80. *Metastasis* of a malignant melanoma

× 135

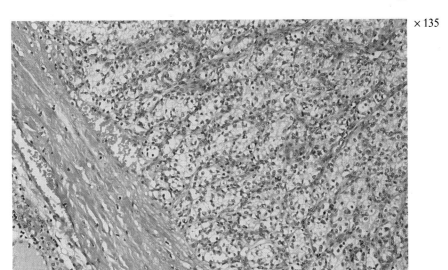

Fig. 81. *Metastasis* of a renal clear cell adenocarcinoma

× 135

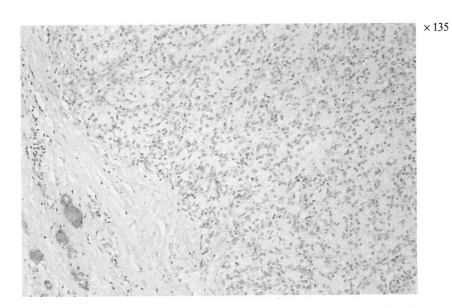

Fig. 82. *Metastasis* of a renal clear cell adenocarcinoma. Same tumour as Fig. 81. Anti-thyroglobulin, positive only in residual follicles

62

× 55

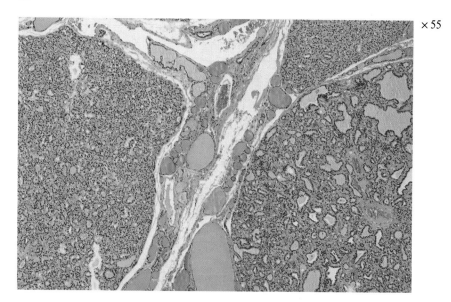

Fig. 83. *Adenomatous goitre*, predominantly microfollicular

× 55

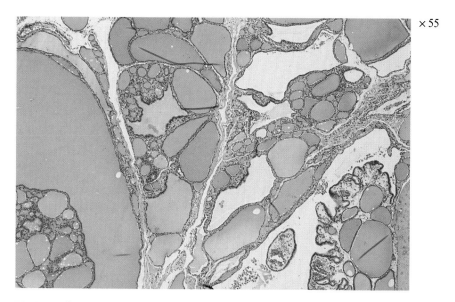

Fig. 84. *Adenomatous goitre*, macrofollicular

×55

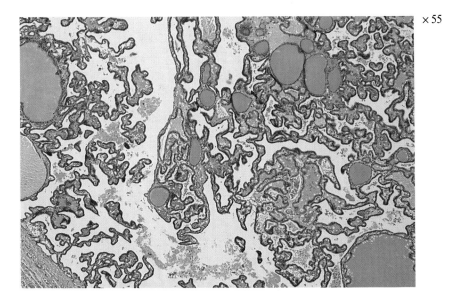

Fig. 85. *Adenomatous goitre,* macropapillary nodule

×135

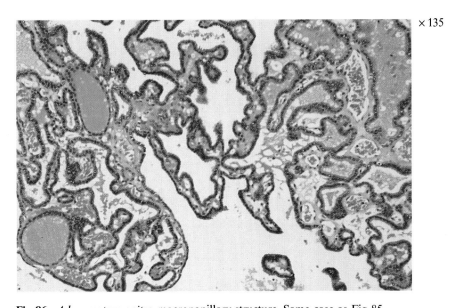

Fig. 86. *Adenomatous goitre,* macropapillary structure. Same case as Fig. 85

64

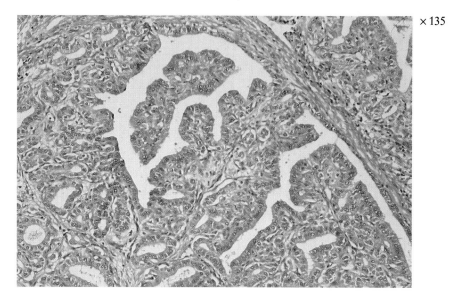

×135

Fig.87. *Hyperplastic goitre* with pseudopapillary formations. Patient with Graves' disease (Basedow's disease)

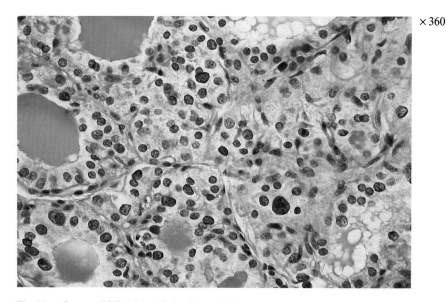

×360

Fig.88. *Abnormal follicular cells.* Patient with Graves' disease (Basedow's disease)

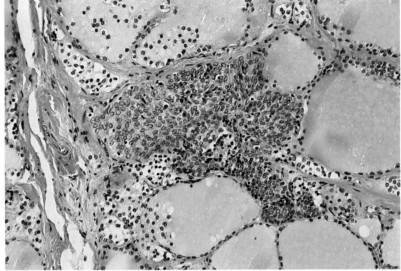

Fig. 89. *Solid cell nest*

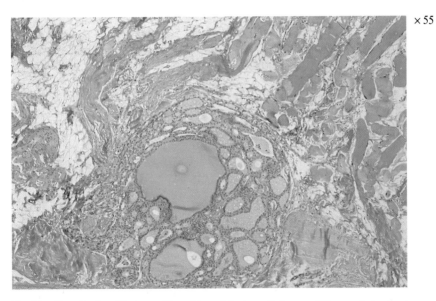

Fig. 90. *Ectopic thyroid tissue.* Thyroid nodule in soft tissue of the neck (patient had been operated for nodular goitre)

66

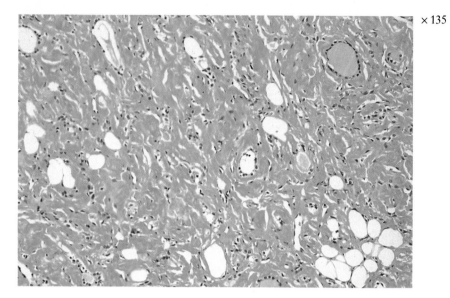

×135

Fig. 91. *Amyloid goitre*

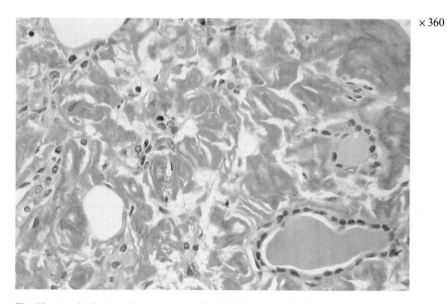

×360

Fig. 92. *Amyloid goitre*. Same case as Fig. 91. Congo Red stain

WHO International Histological Classification of Tumours
Hedinger et al.: Histological Typing of Thyroid Tumours, 2nd edn.

35 mm Color Transparencies

A set of 92 color slides (35 mm), corresponding to the photomicrographs in this book, is available from the American Registry of Pathology. To order these *slides,* send the following information to:

American Registry of Pathology
14th Street and Alaska Ave. NW
Washington, DC 20306 USA

Please send me:

_____ set(s) of 35 mm slides of Histological Typing of Thyroid Tumors at $ 50.00 per set.
For Air Mail outside of North America add $ 10.00.

Total cost: $ _____ .00

Name _____

Address _____

_____

_____

Date _____ Signature _____

☐ I enclose a check/money order in US$ payable to the ARP.
☐ Please charge my credit card:
    ☐ VISA
    ☐ MasterCard

Card number _____

Expiration date _____

Name as it appears on credit card _____

Prices are subject to change without notice.

International Union Against Cancer

P. Hermanek, L. H. Sobin (Eds.)

TNM Classification of Malignant Tumors

4th, fully revised edition. 1987.
XVIII, 197 pages. Soft cover.
ISBN 3-540-17366-8

The TNM System is the most widely used classification of the extent of growth and spread of cancer. This revised, unified, fourth edition of the TNM Classification is published as the result of a joint venture by the American, British, Canadian, French, German, Italian and Japanese National TNM Committees.
The new edition eliminates all variations, up-dates existing site classifications and adds chapters on previously unclassified tumours.

Springer-Verlag
Berlin Heidelberg New York
London Paris Tokyo

B. Spiessl, O. H. Beahrs,
P. Hermanek, R. V. P. Hutter,
O. Scheibe, L. H. Sobin,
G. Wagner (Eds.)

TNM-Atlas

Illustrated Guide to the TNM/$_p$TNM Classification of Malignant Tumours

3rd edition. 1988. Approx.
452 figures. Approx. 350 pages.
ISBN 3-540-17721-3

The present third edition of the TNM Atlas is based on the fourth edition of the internationally unified TNM Classification of Malignant Tumours, that was accepted by all national TNM Committees, including the American Joint Committee on Cancer, and was enlarged by previously unclassified tumours. The TNM Atlas follows the sound principles of the previous editions and comprises numerous illustrations to visualize the anatomical extent of malignant tumours at the different stages of their development. It is designed as an aid for the practical application of the TNM Classification for all doctors working in the field of oncology.

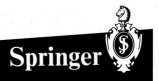

Springer